DENTAL ETIQUETTE
Externship Tips
For Dental Assistants

A preparation Guide for Dental Assistants
1st Edition

Theresa Biggs RDA, CDA, Dental Instructor

Don't Let This Be You!

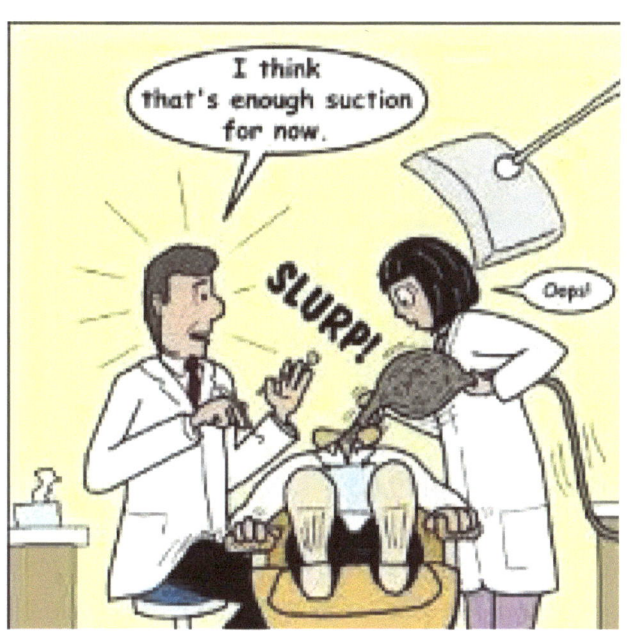

Preface

The bridge from completing your dental assistant program to transitioning to the actual dental field can be scary and sometimes your just not prepared enough for what you could encounter your first day as an Assistant that you worked hard to get to with long homework assignments with taking impressions over and over until you master the lip roll and knowing your instruments. So much goes into training an assistant but what do you do when you encounter problems at the new office or what is expected of you the first day is sometimes vague to new assistants. This book is written for all new dental assistants getting ready to face the Dental world and give you a full panoramic view of your steps to be gainfully employed by a DDS you want to work for and not just settle for so you can blossom like a caterpillar into a Butterfly! You can achieve your dreams within this Health Industry with the knowledge of others, including but not limited to myself who has worked in this field since 1991.

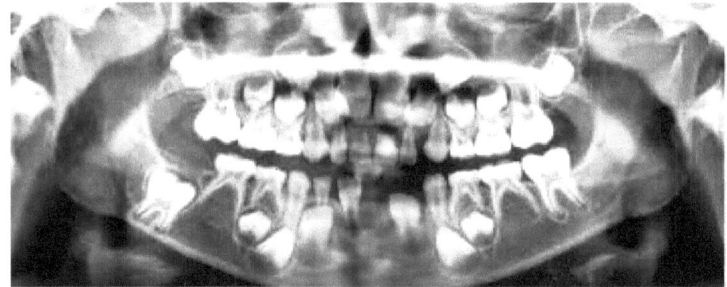

The Panoramic view is to see yourself not just in school but as well as succeeding in any part of dentistry you apply yourself to from Dental Floater to EFDA even an Office Manager! Yes you can wear different hats in this field and it is better to be cross trained and keep adding to your skills by continuing to learn as you go and saving important things along your way. Dental Assistant Textbooks are great for learning the skills you need to learn but there are Dental Etiquette skills which is the customary code of polite behavior in society or among members of your profession you must learn before entering this field. Let's begin your journey together with this book where you will get first hand inside to my personal and professional experience in this field to help you be one of those assistants the doctor needs to have by their side during those tough procedures.

Just like the Panorex above gives a panoramic view of the entire patients mouth it is also a great example of how some offices have assistants who are pushed out of their position by another assistant or some make room for the next generations of assistants while new positions are formed within the office just like Wisdom teeth erupt where no present teeth are present or being pushed out like a permanent tooth pushing a primary tooth out so is this field so please take note of what is expected of you so you will be either the wisdom tooth or the permanent tooth and not staying just primary in your new career!

> **If there's a Will, there's a Way**

EXPLANATION OF EXTERNSHIP

The externship provides Dental Assistant students with learning opportunities from actual experience with establish Dental professionals who share their knowledge with the new generations of Dental Assistants

Example

Dental Office Manager Working At Externship Office Your At Has **20** Years Experience and not just at the office their at now.

Dental Assistant Currently Employed at office has worked there for 12 years but has 5 years experience somewhere else. Total experience **17** years

Dental Assistant #2 has **1** year experience

Dental Hygienist has **4** years of experience at same office

Dental Hygienist (Fill in) has **14** years experience

Dentist has **35** years of experience from education to running a practice!

Total years of experience and knowledge you are learning from during externship if you were at this office would be **87** years of Day to Day knowledge you can learn from so most importantly take the site your at with approaching it with Respect because they are established already and you are seeking employment soon and they could and would be a reference for you if not a possible hiring opportunity within the company or Dentistry is a small world and Dentist do talk to their peers and they might very well have a colleague who is looking for a new staff member.

First Impressions-Your Resume

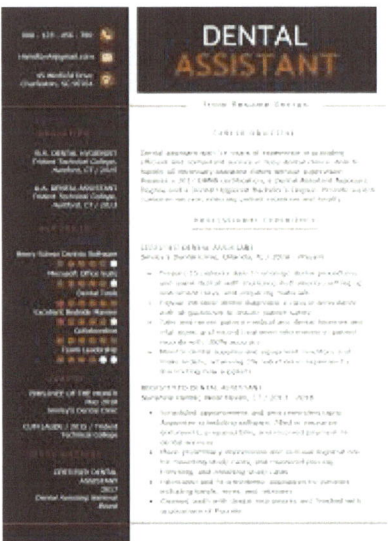

Amazon Kindle Readers Can Click Teachable Link Below To Take You To Purchase My Resume Outline To Help You Write Up A Resume To Stand Out. Price $25.00 Don't worry Hard Copy Readers Just Type In This Link
https://dental-assisting-course.teachable.com/p/mini-course-template

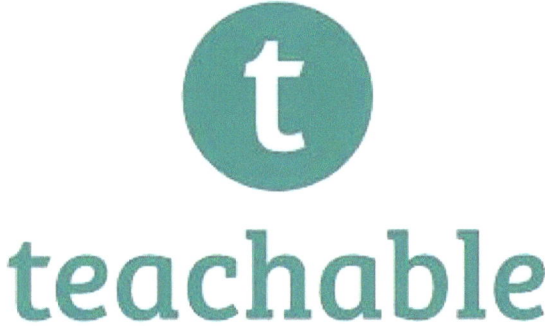

The first thing you must prepare is a Resume to have to give to the externship site either for participation of your externship or exiting it for future hires at their office.

Resumes should have all the basics from the Name to Education and Employment History but what is it on their that would make you stand out and give you more experience in the process? Well I know and I am sharing a few of my little secret that has helped many of my students who have applied for it! The rest can be found on my site this is so I can stay focused on Externship in this book.

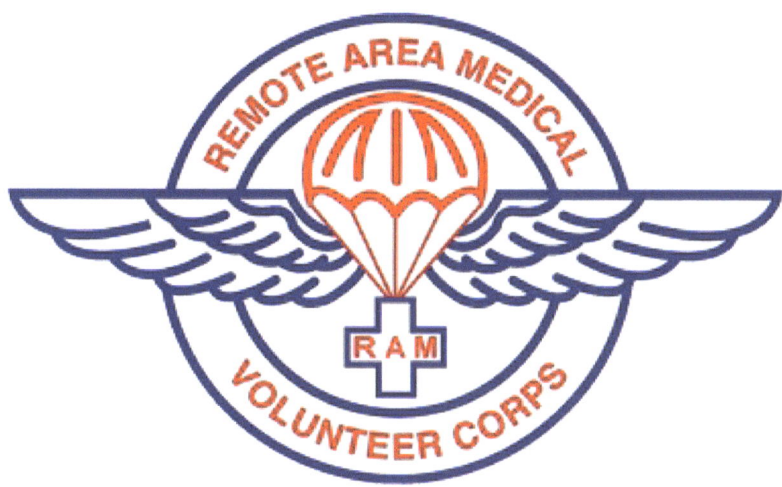

Apply To Volunteer with Remote Area Medical
Will lead to but not limited to….
- Gaining Experience To Add To Resume
- Meeting Fellow Dental Professionals within you community
- Can Have it on Resume Right after you sign up
- Shows you are dedicated
- Shows you care for patients even the non paying ones!
- Leads To Employers who are hiring

Ready To Apply
I am adding Link https://www.ramusa.org/

Most Dental Practitioners want someone who is ready to take over a position or even be a lead assistant at an office that has only one assistant! Did you know you could find yourself being the only one there to do all the jobs as a Dental Assistant? Are you ready? If not don't panic but apply what you have learned already and don't stop there you must continue to learn as you go in this field and you will make mistakes and learn from them, hopefully the first time you make the mistakes because some professionals frown upon having to tell you to do something more than once. So While they are showing you ASK questions! Don't be intimidated or feel you already know it all but this individual is taking time out to teach you something so show them your listening by asking questions don't be a deer in headlights!

Externship can lead to Employment I first hand have seen many students get hired even while on Extern because they walked into the office knowing their hands on skills.
You want to stand out among your fellow classmates as well as many other assistants from neighboring schools

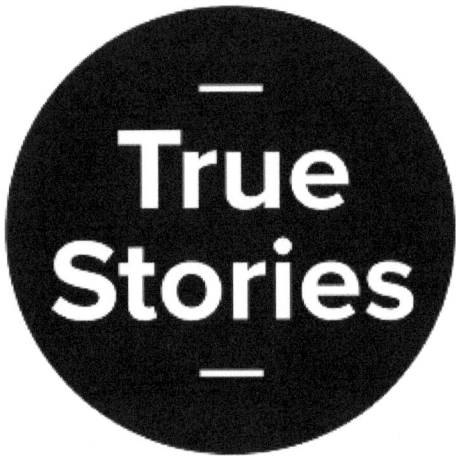

You will be surprised to learn that even your actions can keep future assistant students from being able to apply their skills behind you if you leave a bad impression. Once you get out there you are an example for not just the school but as well as for your Instructors you had along the way.

I once was told by an Orthodontist his frustrations of externship students coming into the office and standing around on their phones while he and his staff are trying to train them in their speciality which is already hard to get your foot in the door for and learning from him and his staff would give those students the abilities to bond brackets, fit bands and everything else you need to know as an Orthodontic assistant.

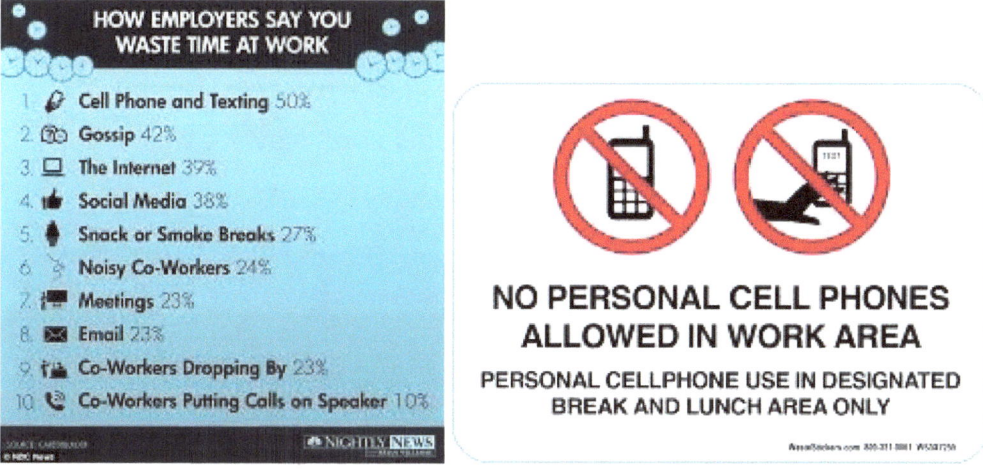

In our discussion he talked about how other students are keeping him from training more students from the same school due to their lack of interest of past students. You do have an impact at your externship and must hold a certain professionalism for this Health care Industry so others may follow along your path to achieve their goals as well. Our conversation was short but understood he wanted to know more about my students and the school I work for because he took some of my students right out of school and was pleased with them that he hired them. I want the same for you and your school to be successful because I do believe in word of mouth and word does get around in this Dental world. Patients are very important as well during your externship and will get into that later in this book.

Let's get into What They Expect of You First Day

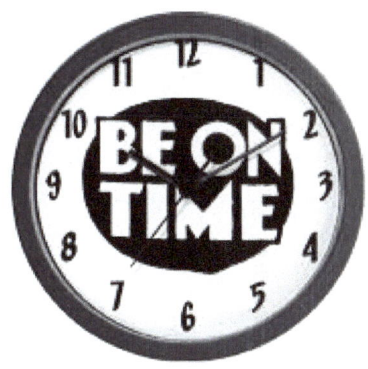
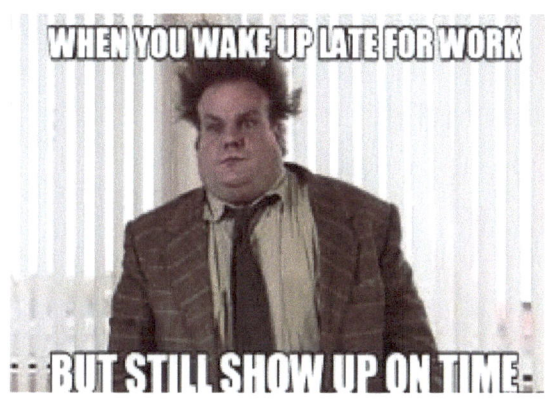

#1 Show up Yes Some don't show up to the first day, Some students miss for a number of reasons and don't even bother calling the school or office they are to be at to explain what happened. I have seen many social media comments about students and interviews no shows and how frustrating that is when the Doctor has to stay on schedule and they are waiting for someone to give them a chance.

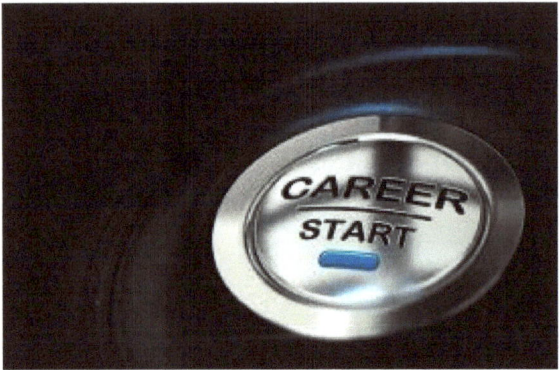

Tips: Do a test drive to the office to see how long it would take you or use google maps to know the right route for that time so you can avoid rush hour which can make you late. Make sure you have gas the day before to save you from stopping in the morning and have to wait in line.

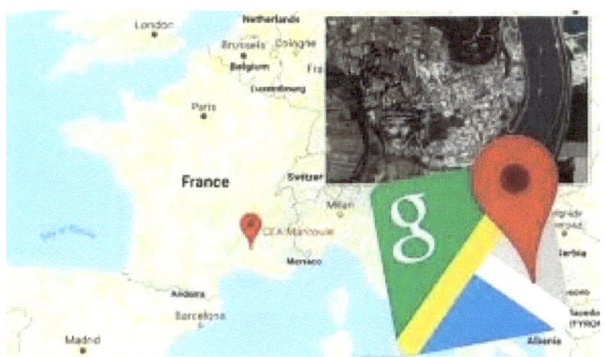

Can use for walking as well

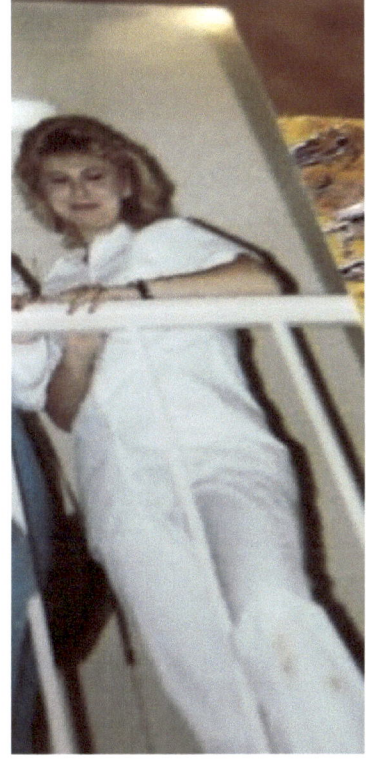

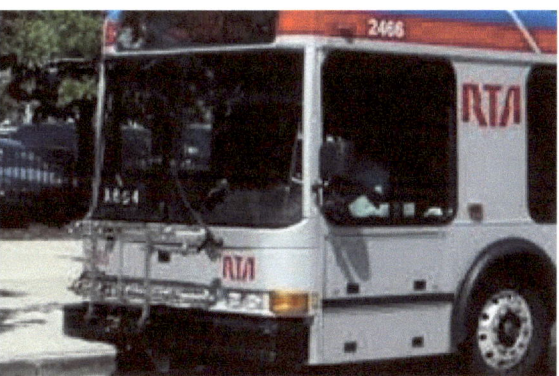

I caught 2 buses to get to school and to my new job and it pays off trust me, you will be on your way to driving if you aren't yet. I would bring extra pants if yours get dirty like mine are above by my knees from snow melting and dirty splashing on them.

#2 Blend In By Looking Professional

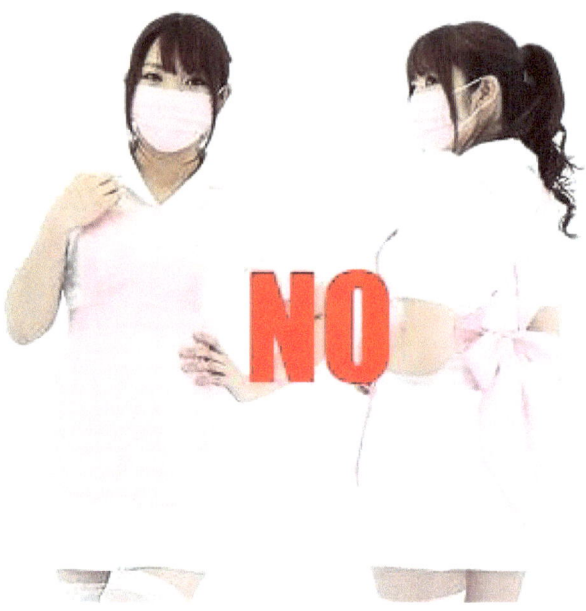

　　Clean Scrubs Not wrinkly or stained up also ask ahead if they prefer you to wear a certain color and if you don't have it go with a neutral color like gray,black,white.

　　Proper shoes and clean don't have to be new but they do have to look like you clean for the office floors are spotless in most places I have seen doctors complain of assistants dragging mud into the office and it is frowned upon.

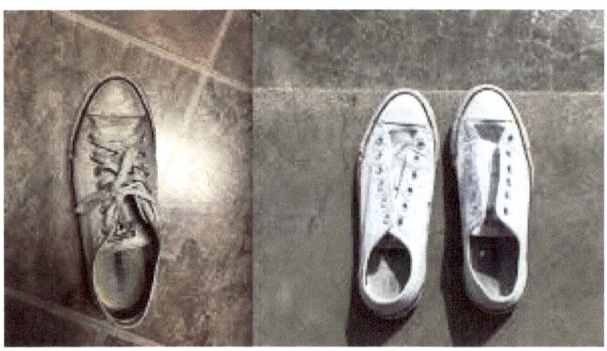

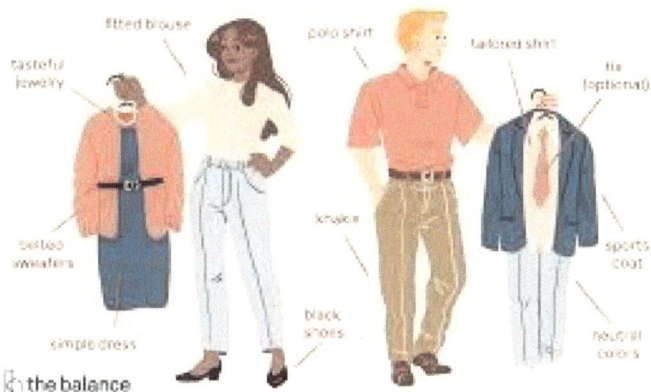

Business Casual Dress for Work

Hair Neat Many offices prefer short hair or if longer hair tied up or out of the way for OSHA reasons. If you love to color while seeking work make sure it is a natural color shade some are just old school and they decide to hire you. I personally the Author of this book was fired once due to coloring my hair from blond to black to look more like my deceased mother and the doctor liked blonds ,So I share this because it is a fact that it does happen but the truth always comes out and there was more to the story which I share in my Dental Affairs Book.

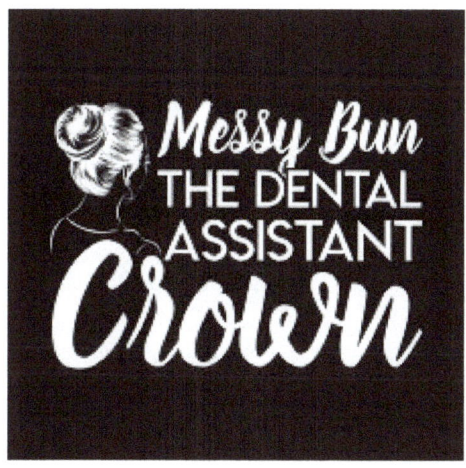

Perfume just a dab or two remember patients can have allergies to it remember less is better because you do work in small treatment areas.

Piercings if at first your going to interviews and not figuring out why your not getting hired. The office has an image they want to uphold and some don't like it because it can affect how their patients see their office and as well as most dental professionals do not like the tongue piercing because it can damage the teeth and how do we educate our patients if we are not setting the example.

Bacteria will get in it and gloves will rip in the middle of procedures.

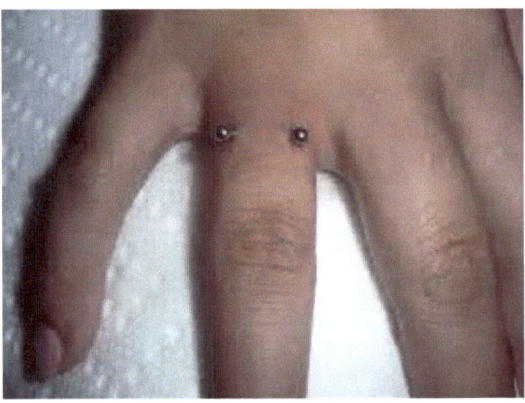

Nails should be short and clean to keep down Germs and according to OSHA standards. Yes we love our nails and some places will allow you to have nails keep in mind you can easily pinch the patients tissue with it.

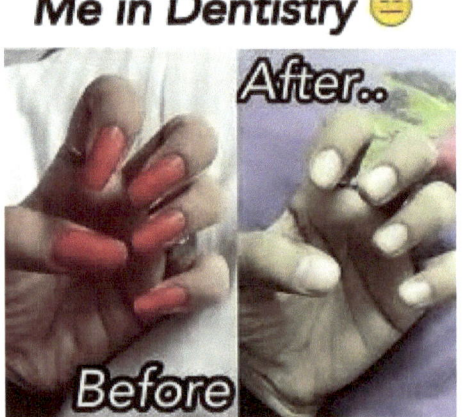

Tattoos unfortunately I have had first hand experience as an instructor with a very good student who kept going on interviews and when she reaches out to me I asked her to nicely asked why she didn't get the position and there it was her tattoo on the back of her neck was causing her not to get hired so she change her hairdo and next thing we know she heard Your Hired! It is their office and some states they have to right to fire for any reason. So if you have any visible tattoos while trying to find employment cover them up. I have seen some places not care but far and few.

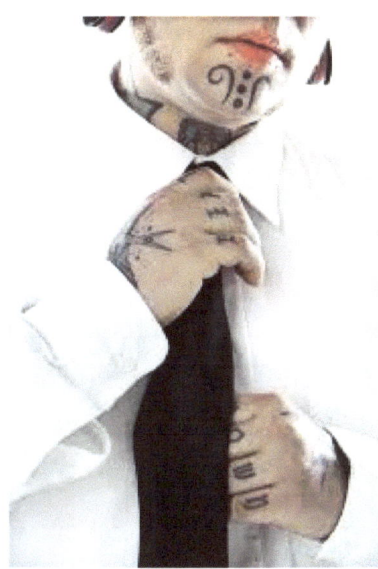

#3 Be Prepared

Eat Make sure you have a good breakfast even if it a snack bar, I have said this time and time again in my classes and there are those ones that are so busy they still forget to eat and my most recent story was one of my A+ students did not eat and she fainted and Dr.McDreamy woke her up and needless to say she was embarrassed about it. Another time I was working at an Orthodontist office running my chair when the new girl just fell over. One more I can think of is I was teaching at one school and explaining the trimming wheel when all of a sudden my student next to me fainted. Please make sure you eat so you have the energy to take care of others. #1 First is you!

Items To Bring

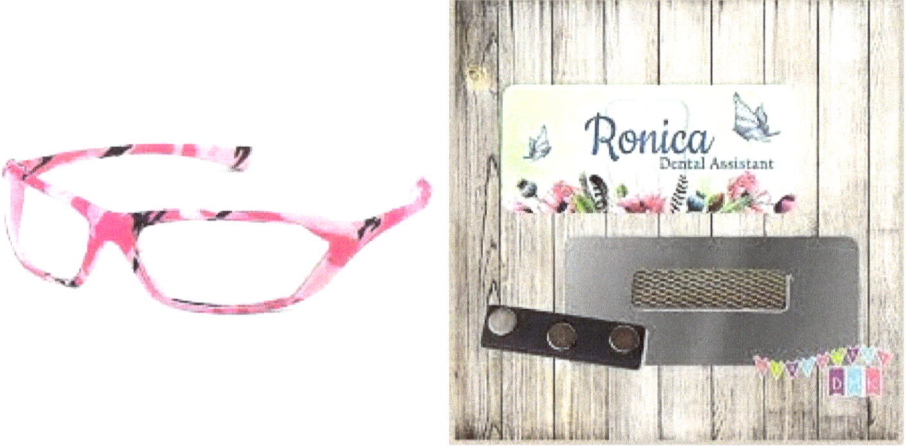

Do you have <u>safety glasses</u> you should have a pair just incase the last assistant walked out with them they don't always have extra. On my website for students I have resources for such things including showing up with your <u>name tag</u> looking the part!
https://dentalindexjr.weebly.com/uniforms-dos--donts.html

Smokers: Reminder Dental professionals who works in close proximity to Fellow staff members and patients should never smell cigarette smoke while on duty. This is rude to some staff members and patients. The smell keeps the office from being a sanitary working environment and does not smell pleasing leaving the office with smokers odor. Plus it is working against your smile which is very important in this field for you are to lead your patients as an example that is why most Dental offices offer free or discounted Dental to their staff as well as some offer free Orthodontics.

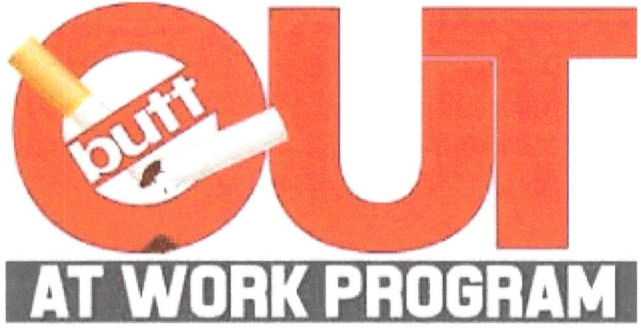

Pack a lunch incase the schedule is running over and you don't want to leave the staff who stays stuck even if your there to help and get the hours you need, keep in mind they take all that into consideration when maybe looking for a new staff member and you are unaware of it or keep you in mind for the future.

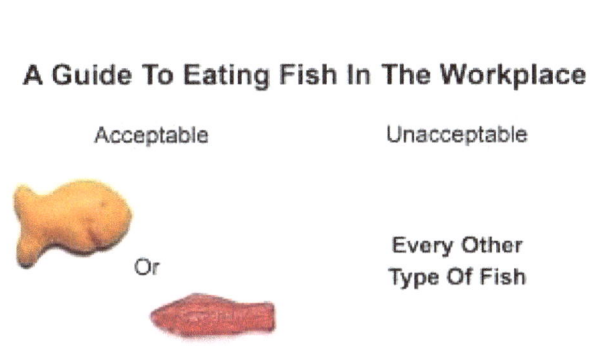
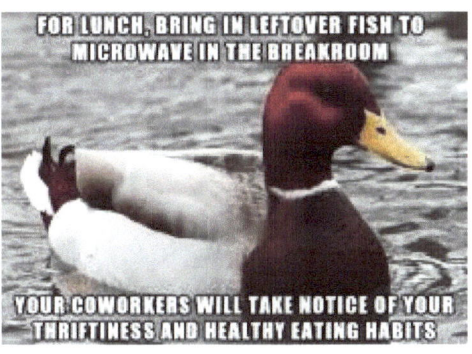

#4 Be Knowledgeable and Ready To Step In!

Never leave in the middle of a procedure it is frowned upon and have everything ready so you don't even have to get up for a paper towel or extra gauze have it out already and if you must go in drawers during procedure use a clean pair of cotton pliers and be sure to close the drawer afterwards. The eyes will be on you to make sure you are following OSHA guidelines because you are under the Doctors supervision by the State and he could get fined for your mistakes.

Please note that know when is perfect and always own up to your mistakes so when a big one happens and you know you didn't do it they can recall how honest you always have been being forthcoming when you did make a mistake.
Note: Good example a Sneeze happens in the middle of working what do you do when Dentist is deeply involved in procedure and you have to either deal with the mess in your mask after the procedure or stop when you can and change mask fast and wash hands reapply gloves of course new ones and then keep on working. It does happen but you don't realize until that moment so thought I add it into this book to warn you ahead of time.

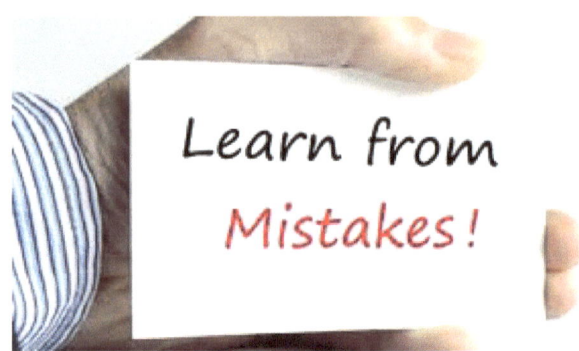

Never laugh at your patients

(It could strike your funny bone at times so put mask over face. Reminder patients can read eyes!) Plus patients don't like when you talk over them about your weekend. They complain to the front or sometimes just leave the practice. Join them in the conversation and keep in mind some don't like to be social don't take it personally you don't know what they have gone through in life to make them that way.

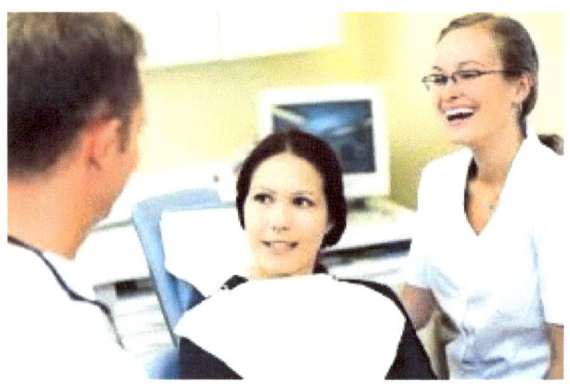

Wear Your PPE Gloves-Mask-Safety Glasses

Never assume the old grandma was't wild in her day or the young child wasn't born with an illness so keep yourself safe. Plus if your carrier for your patients safety as well.

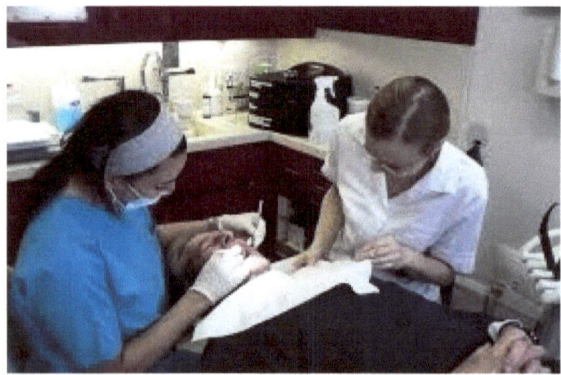

Avoid Office Gossip

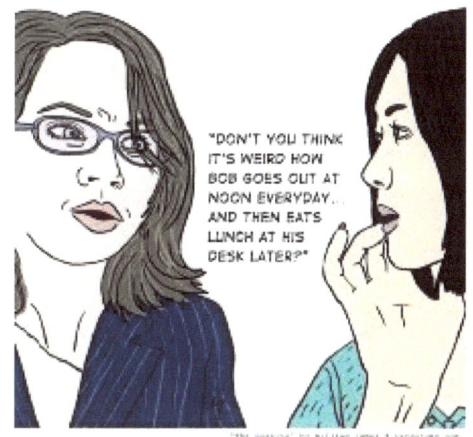 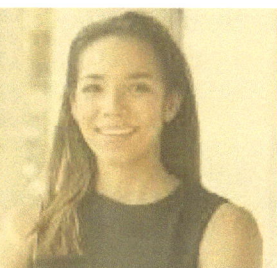

You could be tested by staff members to see if you join their click or they are seeing if you are a troublemaker. Just stay clear of it. Period. Keep in mind that treatment rooms are thin and sound travels.

Posture
Yes postures is important because it reflects your confidence level and your Interest in your new career also your attitude speaks volumes in a small office it can be picked up easily.

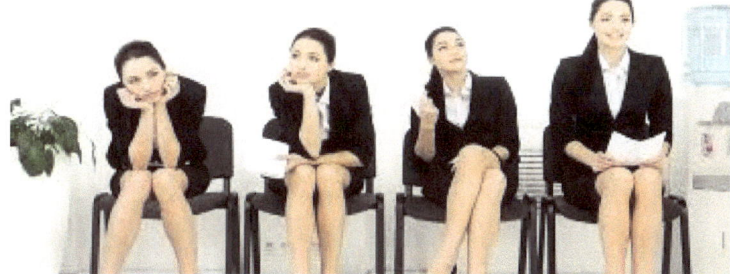
Don't slouch

A Negative attitude can often lead a person to slouch as well as hurt your body because it can become habit forming.

Verbal Manners
Tone

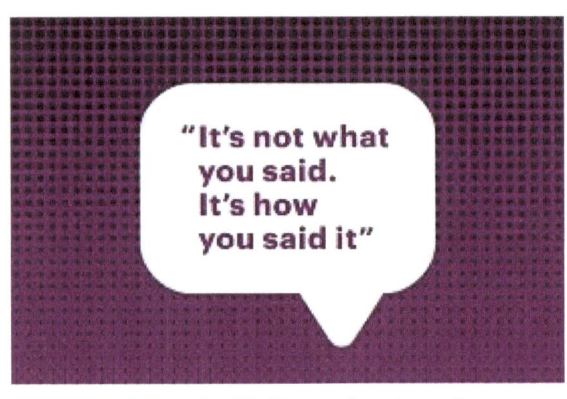
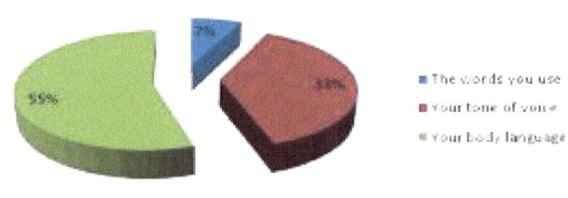

Choice of words: Talk professionally
You never want to say Huh? What? Instead say Excuse me? Pardon me?
Here is an oldie but goodie when you say Yah instead say yes
Or Nah say no
I ain't did that instead instead say I did not

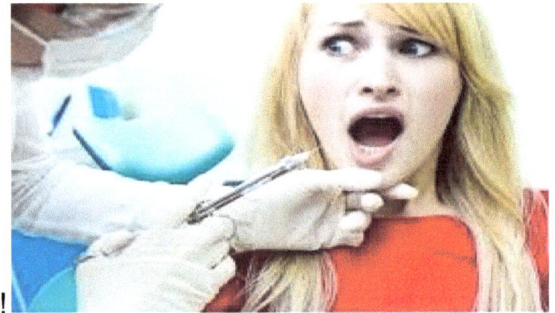

And don't say most of all Yah Doc I got the shot!

Words To Avoid	Say Instead
Renew	Expire
Cheap	Less expensive
Quote/Bid	Proposal
Best deal	Better value
Pitch	Presentation
Truthfully/Honestly/Trust me	I'm confident that …
Contract	Agreement
Sign	Ok
Customer	Client

Sounds

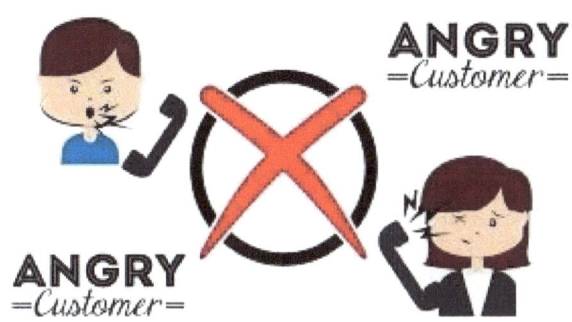

Now when a patient is upset remember it could be for more than other reasons at hand if they are short temper so be sure to speak calmly and address the issue with the Dentist without bringing the Dentist to front if at all possible try to handle the situation yourself but if patient wants answers let them know you understand their concern and you will do your best to get to a solution. Let them know and hear it in your voice a person who keeps yelling will calm down to hear your low voice that is speaking calmly to them and will reflect on their own behavior.

Note: If Dentist is working on a patient and it is a matter that can not wait then write it on a sticky note and show them, Have a pen ready incase they have to write something down to tell you so other patient in chair doesn't hear it.

Social Behavior

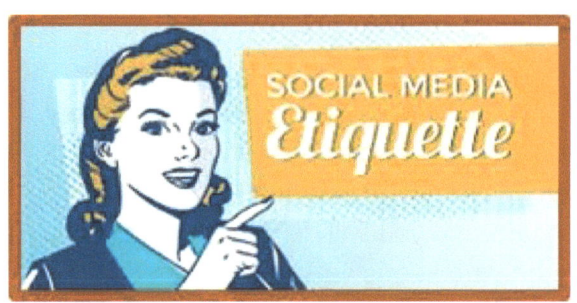
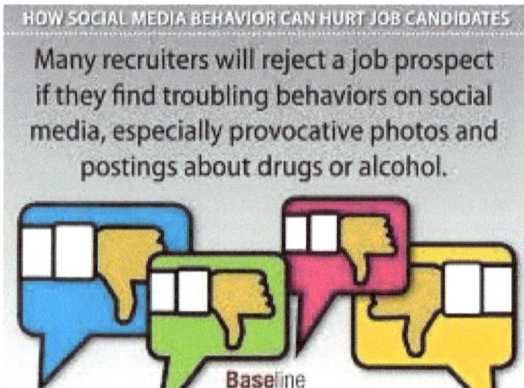
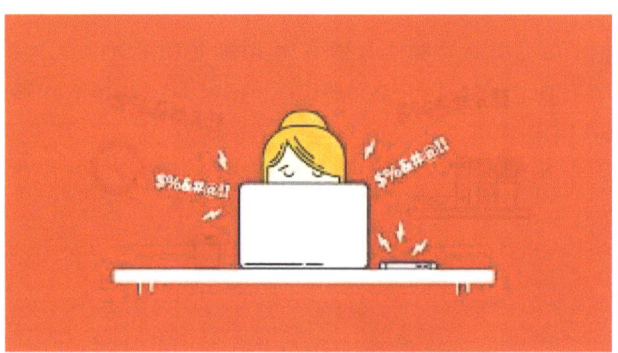

Watch what you are posting it can be rude or offensive to others as well as damaging to finding work. I have read so many negative posts on Youtube, Facebook, especially in the groups which I use to encourage my students to join but as an Instructor I want my students to be a certain way and I started getting feedback from my students of the negative comments they were reading and it is one thing to deal with your own office issues let alone unlimited problems on social media and everyone has some type of feedback and I notice so many are ready to criticize other DA's instead of helping, I share this because my small voice might make a change for more positive assistants out there so before you decide to join the complaints of many others there is always a solution to an issue, If you have a fellow Dental Professional who is giving you a hard time just ask them with keeping your composer always because someone might be around the corner listening as I have seen others up against a wall trying to listen in an office at times. Yes as crazy as it sounds a work family has its moments so be sure you keep clear just stay clear from drama day 1 if you find yourself in an office like this. I have had my share of others telling me don't work so hard you make us look bad. Here it is you look out for your Employer and Yourself and be the best Co-worker you would want to have next to you goes back to that old but good saying "Treat others how you want to be treated" Let this new

Generations of Assistants outshine and that is what we all should want just like raising kids we want them to do better than we have done at least we should.
Call me the GodMother of Dental Assistants because I care truly care about this career because what you teach others who are going to care for others to me well that is just so important beyond words.

Happy Doctor+Happy Co-Workers+Happy You= Happy Work Environment and Patients pick up on it.

Or it could be this way

Unhappy You being negative rubs off on Unhappy Doctor which in turns out the whole staff is miserable.

Bottomline They will check Social Media to see who you are as you should as well and check out there website and be ready to let them know you did to learn their office and Doctors Education Background.

Let your light Shine and Bring Joy to others and if it drains you Refuel with a hobby or Family Time. Something outside work so you don't get burned out.

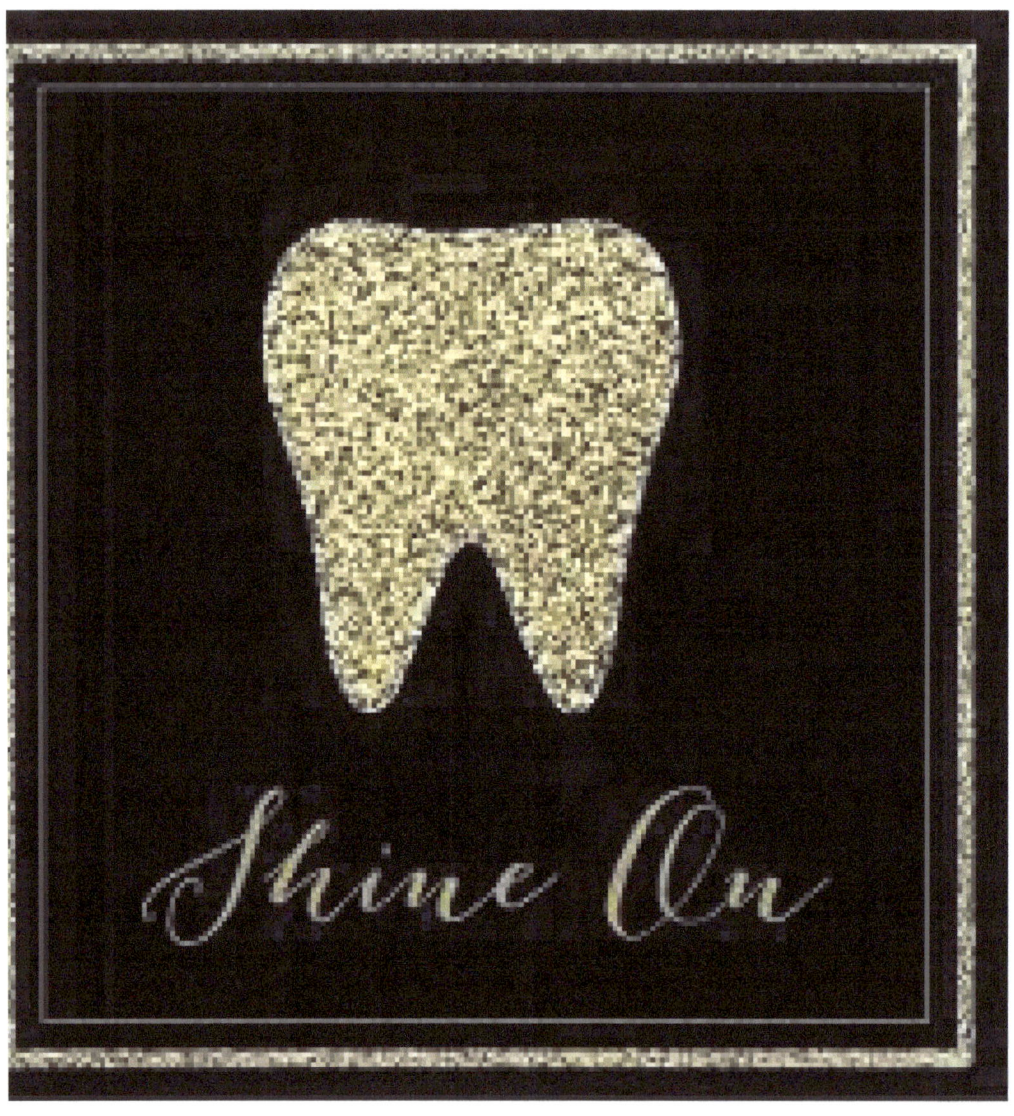

First Day Scenario

They will greet you and show you around and some places might let you get right to work while some Dentist might ask you to observe at first but keep in mind Externship is for getting your hands in those gloves and working all day as if it was a job you are getting paid for also sharing the load with the team. Introduce yourself to patients because They will give their opinion to The Dentist and as I mentioned earlier, patients are very important because if no patients then slow day if a slow day then most likely have to go home. So be sure to interact with the patients and remember to use vaseline for the corner of their lips so they don't wake up with cracked lips and put some on a gauze with a topical applicator which will help you apply it and explain while you are and watch it shows right off the bat you care. Offer a blanket to the patients and if the office has a neck pillow offer that.

Who wants to be in a Dental chair and feel exposed laying there which is where the blanket helps. If you start at an office and they don't do this then suggest it! Some patients are friends with the doctor and they will call them later to talk to them during a post op call which is calling the patient the next day to see how they feel and no not every office does this which most love it when we call and ask so if your DDS doesn't have time to do so then offer that.

You should also become familiar with where things are and most places they set up the rooms all the same so be sure to check with lead assistant if you can look around. Also ask what kind of Dental software they use and don't forget I have Free Tutorials on my website. https://dentalindexjr.weebly.com/dentrix.html This link will lead you to the other programs I found free training on!

You will be given a time sheet to keep track of your hours at some schools and must get it filled out and share with your school if required. You can always ask the Doctor how are you doing and ask them what can you approve on because this is still your time for learning and we all started somewhere so they understand and it shows your interest.

Here is my favorite because I have taught many and have learned different schools do teach differently but never point at someone for not training you in this or that or blame it on your Instructor because they could have shown it and former students were capable of doing the same procedure. Plus it is just tacky so refrain from blame and just realized you didn't learn it but guess what you are now in the office at that moment! Which brings me to the next point take notes! Have a little notepad in your pocket and write notes when ungloved and during slow time to recall what you learned that day. I will enclose a few additional sheets for you in this book to write down what you learned at each office you are doing your extern at.

HIPAA must be followed when writing notes don't write patient names for any reason to protect the privacy act and if you see anyone you know at the site from your day to day world or someone from the past be sure not to break HIPAA then as well talking to others that you saw so and so there at your site.

Knock knock..
Who is there
 HIPAA..
HIPAA Who?
Sorry Can't Tell You! LOL

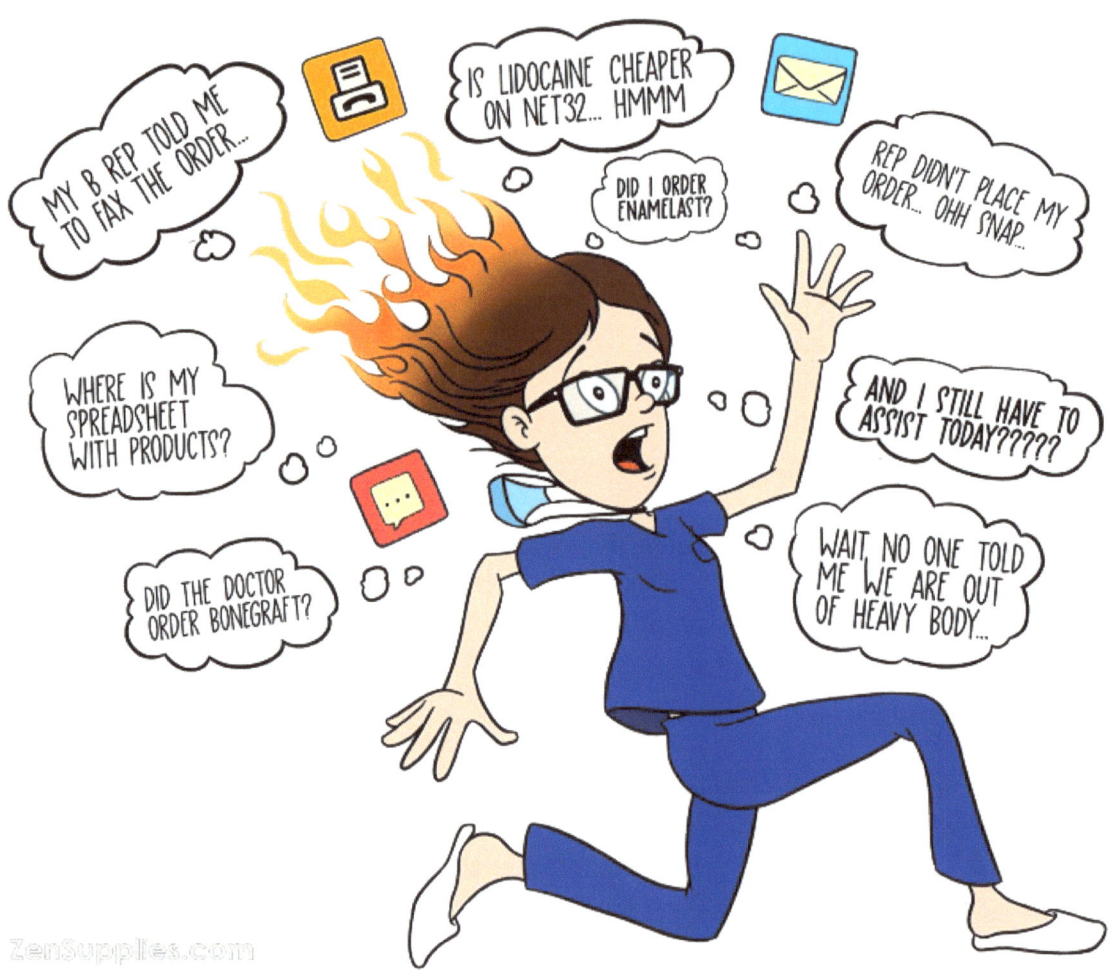

When your done at the Site be sure to follow up with a Thank you letter or Card to give to Dentist and staff for showing you the ropes and leave a lasting reminder because they could be called for your future job or maybe they might offer you one!
I wish you the Best in your New Career and Don't be so hard on yourself you will forever keep learning as for myself I still am learning each day new things.
Embrace Your Journey

Other Books By Author Theresa Biggs RDA,CDA Dental Instructor

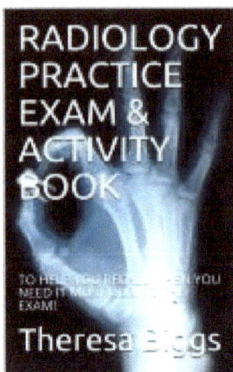

https://amzn.to/2QMsZcE

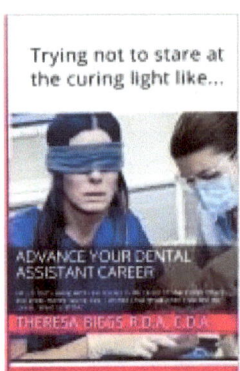

https://amzn.to/2QTHc7w

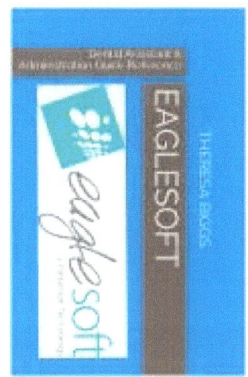
https://amzn.to/35yq1MS

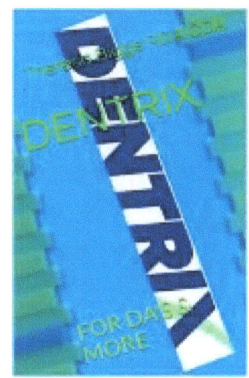
https://amzn.to/2Ofb2ls

www.ingramcontent.com/pod-product-compliance
Lightning Source LLC
Chambersburg PA
CBHW051830210526
45473CB00005B/1818